Sex Vouchers For Her

I0417445

J.L. Silver

Copyright © 2016 J.L. Silver

All rights reserved.

ISBN:10: 1523992816
ISBN-13: 978-1523992812

Eat Me Out Anytime

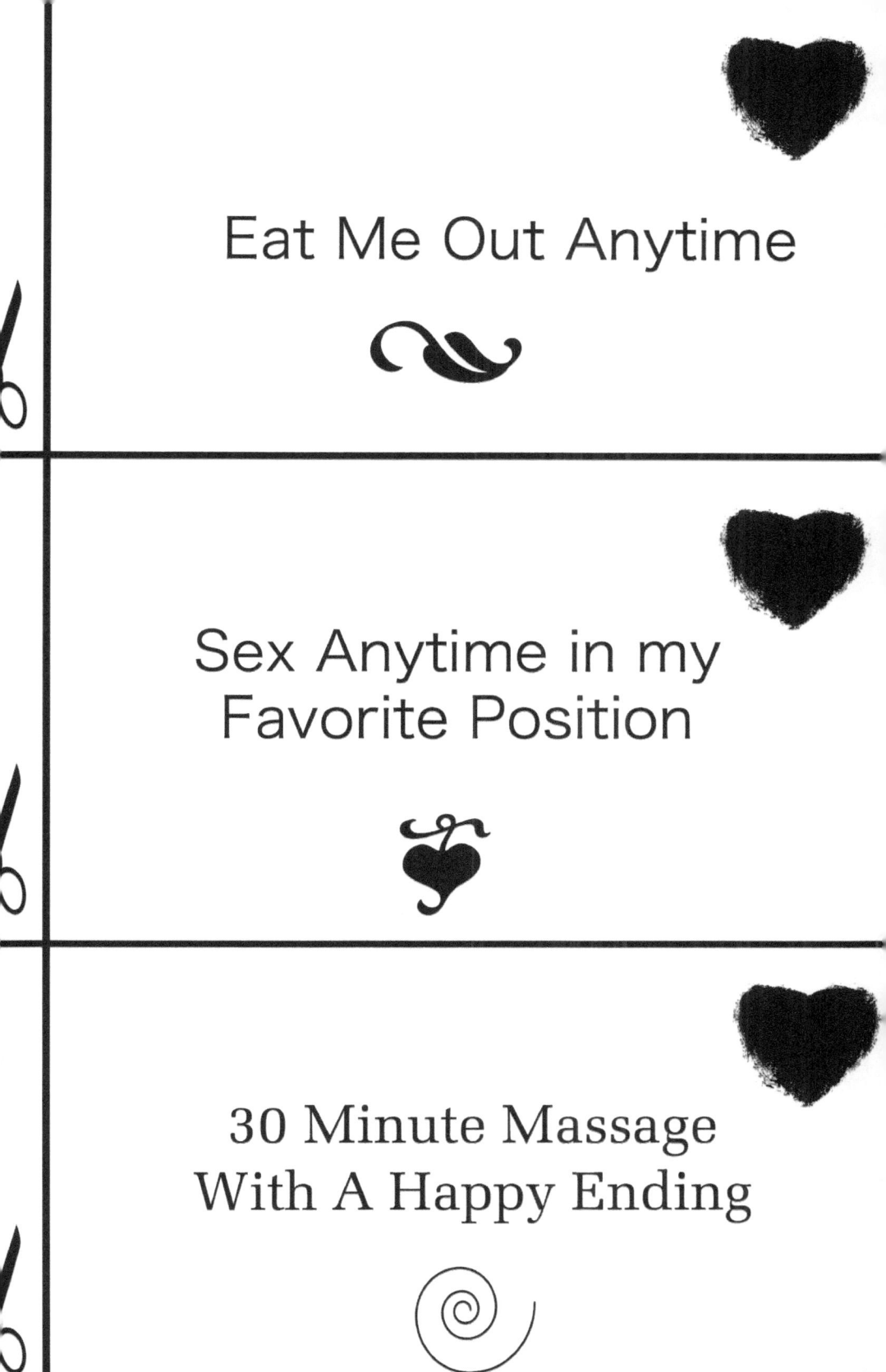

Sex Anytime in my
Favorite Position

30 Minute Massage
With A Happy Ending

Backside of Coupon

Backside of Coupon

Backside of Coupon

Oral Pleasure In The Morning

Doggystyle Sex

Be My Sex Slave For the Night

Backside of Coupon

Backside of Coupon

Backside of Coupon

Eat Me Out At Lunch

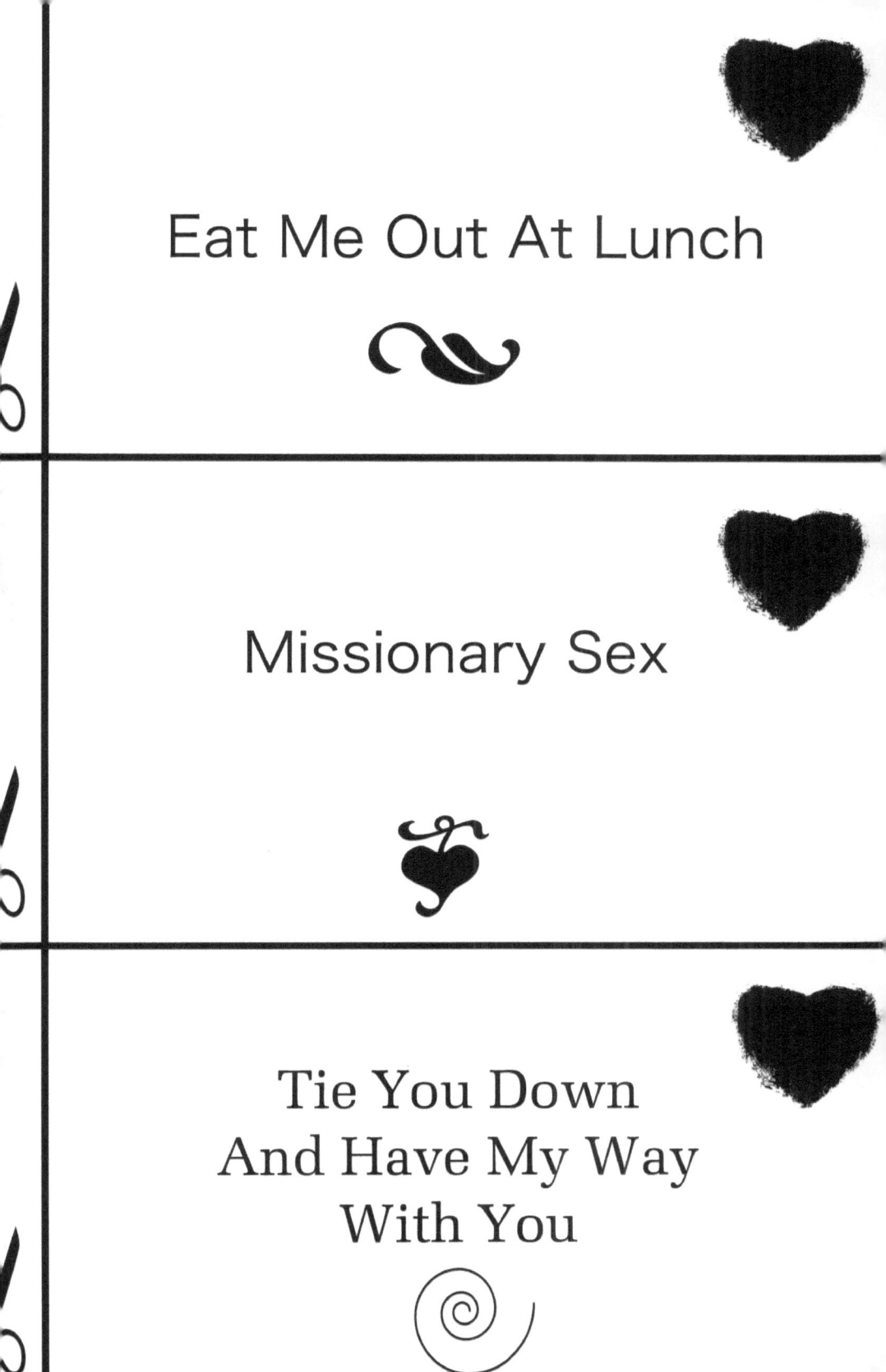

Missionary Sex

Tie You Down
And Have My Way
With You

Backside of Coupon

Backside of Coupon

Backside of Coupon

Go down on me
after work

Reverse Cowgirl

Tie to Chair
And Have My Way
With You

Backside of Coupon

Backside of Coupon

Backside of Coupon

Orally Pleasure Me In The Middle Of The Night

Cowgirl On The Floor

Use A Vibrator on my G-spot and clitoris

Backside of Coupon

Backside of Coupon

Backside of Coupon

Eat Me Out In The Shower

Sex In The Shower

Sex while in
A whirl pool spa
bubble bath

Backside of Coupon

Backside of Coupon

Backside of Coupon

Fuck Me While
Watching A Movie

Sex while I am
in a sex costume

Fuck me on the
washing machine

Backside of Coupon

Backside of Coupon

Backside of Coupon

Eat me out while I play
video games or read a book

Experimental Sex
Try Something New
(Anal, Bondage, etc..)

I will lay down on my
stomach and you
will finger me until
I Cum

Backside of Coupon

Backside of Coupon

Backside of Coupon

69

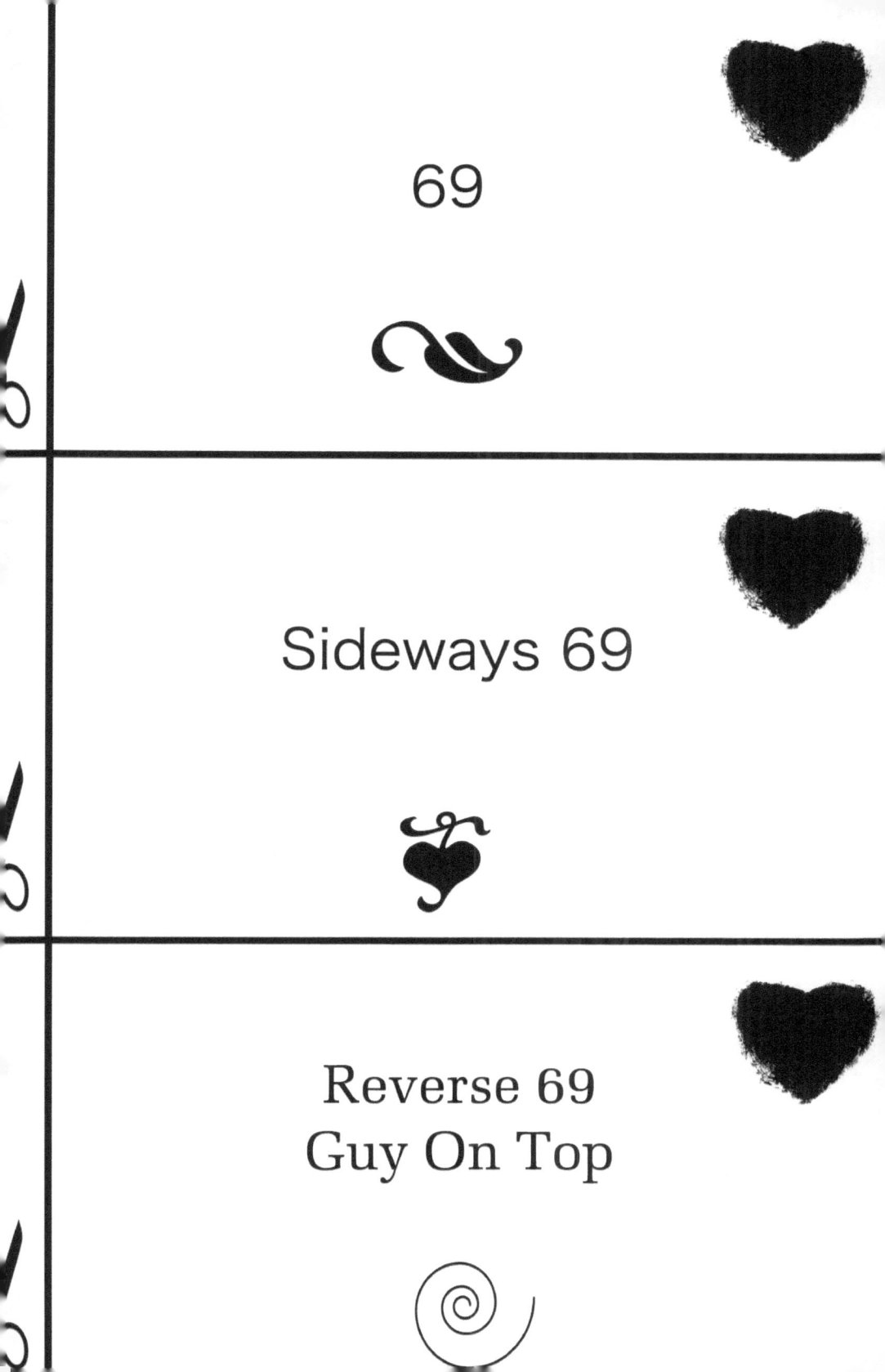

Sideways 69

Reverse 69
Guy On Top

Backside of Coupon

Backside of Coupon

Backside of Coupon

Have him lay at the edge of
the bed with his tongue out
and she will grind on his tongue
until orgasm

he gives you a
striptease

Photoshoot, You direct
him into sexy poses

Backside of Coupon

Backside of Coupon

Backside of Coupon

Have Her lay down on the couch
and he must eat her
out, while she watchs
her favorite show

Masterbate in front
of Me

Make a sex tape
anything goes

Backside of Coupon

Backside of Coupon

Backside of Coupon

Finger my G-spot
And Make me squirt

Tie me down to the bed
and fuck my brains
out

For one week we must
have sex in the when we
get up and when we go to bed.

Backside of Coupon

Backside of Coupon

Backside of Coupon

www.ingramcontent.com/pod-product-compliance
Lightning Source LLC
Chambersburg PA
CBHW021347310526
45786CB00020B/1999